Sirtfood Diet Recipes

Easy, Delicious, and Healthy Sirtfood Cookbook Guide to the Revolutionary New Weight Loss Diet. Burn Fat, Lose Weight, Get Lean, and Feel Great! 7-day meal plan

By Thomas O'Neal

2

Contents

Introduction

Who knew that a diet named Sirtfood would become the new buzzword for the year? Well, as much as the word sirtfood sounds completely unique and different, the diet itself has been surprising people around the world due to its amazing health benefits. In this cookbook, we shall delve deeper into the idea the of sirtfood diet. Where does it get its name from? What is the science behind sirtfood, and who should really be looking out for this diet? These are some of the questions that will be discussed in this cookbook, along with a variety of sirtfood recipes.

Chapter 1

What Are the Sirtfoods?

Even the idea of a sirtfood diet is comparatively new to all, and people are still working to unearth the great mysteries of this diet and find a relation between sirtfood and good health. But so far, much has been learned about the diet through the experts: nutritionists and all the people who have practically tried and tested this diet plan. The word sirtfood is short for sirtuin food. This means that this diet ensures food which is high in sirtuins. What are sirtuins? Well, to be precise sirtuins are proteins that are present in several food items and inside the human body, these proteins can regulate human metabolism, help in weight loss, prevent aging, etc. The important role sirtuins can play in human health has recently been highlighted by most experts and now through the success of the sirtfood diet.

The first book about the sirtfood diet came out in 2016 in the UK, which led to a debate about the effectiveness of this approach. Soon afterward, people started testing this new diet and when Adele premiered with her lean and trim figure in the Billboard Music Awards ceremony, the sirtfood diet got most of the attention. Adele's trainer later revealed how the sirtfood diet really helped the star lose 30 pounds.

Soon after, there appeared many other famous people with their take on the success of this diet. The first-ever text on the diet helped people understand how it can burn fat and prolong a healthy life.

What are Sirtuins?

To know exactly how the sirtfood diet works, it is imperative to understand the role of sirtuins in the human body. In fact, sirtuins are known for playing an important metabolic role in most living organisms. This is why the production, utilization, and stimulation of sirtuins is now considered healthy.

In simple words, sirtuins by their composition are a type of protein present in various parts of the human cell from the nucleus to mitochondria. They are part of the genetic makeup and help in DNA repair and other cell regulation activities.

Sirtuins are also often called the "skinny genes" because of the role they can play in reducing human weight. But how these genes can make that magic happen is an important question. Biological sciences are no magic, it's all about understanding your body better and then meeting the body's needs to help boost its natural healthy activities. Similarly, when we boost the formation and stimulation of sirtuins in the cell, it automatically aids metabolism, prevents aging, and puts the body on a fast track.

Not every person is obese due to lack of exercise or the food they eat—some people have a naturally low metabolic rate and it makes it almost impossible for them to get out of the trap of obesity. By stimulating the sirtuins, we can put the body on track and make burning calories faster and use them effectively.

Who Should Try the Sirtfood Diet?

Anyone who can make the best use out of this diet should try it. There is no one formula of who should try the sirtfood diet and who shouldn't. However, based on the body's needs and the physical problems a person is suffering from, we can decide on a better utility of this diet. Following are the cases in which the sirtfood diet can prove to be most effective.

1. Obesity

Sirtuin burns fats quickly, and that's what makes this diet a great help for weight loss. When we study all the cases of the successful sirtfood dieters, we can clearly see how well they fought against obesity. Adele is just one example, who has amazed the world with her 30 pounds of weight loss achievement using the sirtfood diet. So, anyone who isn't able to lose some extra pounds for whatever reason, they can switch to sirtfood and then can see the magic happening.

2. Low or Poor Metabolic Activity

Since sirtuins are mainly responsible for better cell metabolism, lower sirtuin levels in the body can hamper the natural cell activities and hinders the metabolism. Poor metabolic activity results in weakening of physical strength, obesity, hormonal imbalance, low enzymic activity, and several other related problems. The sirtfood diet is therefore suggested to boost the metabolic rates in the body and revitalize the body and the mind with levels of energy.

3. No workouts

Extraneous workouts are just not for everybody. Sure, working out is a good way to lose some pounds but it is not possible for every other person to invest the required time and energy into the workouts. Therefore, the sirtfood diet can be used by such individuals. Through this diet, they can manage their weight and lose it even while doing some basic physical activities.

4. Aging

Aging seems like a threat to all when those wrinkles start appearing on the skin, and the person feels weakened inside out! Well, this magic gene sirtuin can also play its part in countering the effects of aging. It helps DNA to prolong its life and also aid in the repair process. Sirtuin is also responsible for apoptosis and leads to the formation of new healthy cells. This is the reason that people who are entering into middle age should consider doing the sirtfood diet so that they could effectively fight the possible signs of aging in the years to come.

5. Inflammation

What appears to be weight gain or metabolic inactivity is mostly connected to inflammation of both cells and organs in most cases. This inflammation is both the result and cause of several health problems. Sirtfood does not only prevent inflammation at cellular levels but effectively prevents it at the tissue and organ level.

6. Stress

There is one added advantage that higher sirtuin levels can guarantee and that is the reduction in stress and depression. Research is still being conducted on the relationship between sirtfood and stress, but sirtuin is that element that can enable quick brain cell recovery and boosts brain activity by getting rid of all the unwanted metabolic waste. Efficient brain functioning then leads to a reduction in stress. So, this sirtfood diet can also help with stress relief.

The Procedure of the Sirtfood Diet

One step at a time! That's what it takes to incorporate sirtfood into your diet. The diet is simple and easy to follow in a sense that it only calls for a few definite steps to take. Firstly, you will need to increase food consumption that is rich in sirtuin, then you will have to follow the phases of the diet as discussed in the next section of this book, plus you will need to add green juices to your daily diet. Here are a couple of steps that must be followed to achieve your weight loss goals on a sirtfood diet:

1. Get the right ingredients

Remember that all this diet asks from you is to increase your sirtuins intake. That can be done only through careful and selective grocery shopping. Prepare a list of the ingredients that contain a high amount of sirtuins and check their utility as per your meal plan. There are certain ingredients like coffee, parsley, red wine, and chocolate, that you can have all the time. So, stock up your kitchen cabinets with these ingredients.

2. Set up the schedule

The sirtfood diet gives you small weight loss targets for each week. In the initial time period, you must prepare a schedule to keep track of your meals, the caloric intake, and the timing of green juices you are consuming in a day. In this way, you will be able to manage the first few days of the diet adoption easily and continue observing body changes and measure your weight to keep track of your pace.

3. Prepare for the first week

In the first week of the sirtfood diet, the dieter must control his caloric intake. Therefore, to avoid any mistakes or confusion, all the high caloric food items should be removed from sight. Stuff your refrigerator only with the food that is appropriate for the sirtfood diet, and keep the juices, fruits, and vegetables ready to use. Instead of planning your meal every other day, make plans for the entire week according to the caloric limitations.

4. Caloric intake

Keep in mind that sirtfood is more about weight loss, so mere sirtuins cannot magically work overnight if you keep consuming more calories than your body can actually burn. Do the math and understand your caloric needs, even when the diet does not restrict you from high caloric intake after the first seven days. Still, you must maintain a strict check on the daily caloric intake to keep the weight in control. Otherwise, it does not take much to regain the lost pounds.

5. Green juices

Green juices are one of the most essential parts of the sirtfood diet. These are your way to detoxification and quick weight loss. Green veggies are full of phytonutrients, minerals, and antioxidants. Having them frequently throughout the day can help boost the metabolism, remove the metabolic waste from the body, and enables the body to metabolize the needed nutrients appropriately. These juices are also great for keeping electrolyte balance in the body.

6. Maintenance

To harness the benefit of this diet or any other diet for that matter, it is imperative to maintain your new dietary routine. Most people abandon the diet as soon as they are an oven with the first two phases of the diet or when they achieve their weight loss goals. And soon, they regain weight and blame the diet for being ineffective, which is far from true. It all depends on how consistently you follow this diet plan.

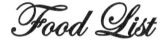

Food List

Sirtuin is found in a wide variety of food that we already consume. But it is the amount of sirtuin that really matters. We can only achieve the health benefits of sirtuin food if we take them frequently and regularly in a perfect amount. Here we have a list of the most common sirtuin-rich food items. It is best to keep them at home and try to use them in different recipes.

1. Dark chocolate

Dark chocolate is a great source of flavonoids, if it is 70% cocoa and unprocessed. It can improve our health in several ways. Even a small piece of this chocolate is a good cure to meet your sugar cravings, and it can also boost the levels of endorphins and serotonin. The chocolate has chemical agents that can also help fight heart diseases, stroke, and high blood pressure.

2. Red wine

It is said that red wine has anti-inflammatory and antioxidant properties, and it can also cure cancer. Red wine is prepared from the skins and seeds of purple grapes. This drink is also rich in polyphenols and resveratrol, and these agents can protect blood vessels from any damage, prevent blood clots, and help to reduce bad cholesterol. One glass of red wine is enough in a day to harness all its benefits, or can be added to your meal in some amount during cooking.

3. Onions

Red onions are not only a low caloric food, and good for flavors, but they can also alleviate the threats of certain cancers, as they have quercetin other than a high amount of sirtuins. Onions are a good source of antioxidants and vitamin C, which naturally boost our immune system.

4. Green tea

Green tea is full of antioxidants that can protect the cells from any damage. Green tea also contains catechins which play its part in increasing natural metabolic rates. Try to use matcha green tea in your daily diet, as it is made with crushed tea leaves, so a small amount of enough to infuse great flavors and lots of nutrients.

5. Blueberries

Blueberries are proven to help in lowering bad cholesterol, successfully fights aging, can cure inflammation, and also aid in fat burning. High in antioxidants and phytonutrients, the blueberries can be enjoyed daily as a snack or in smoothies.

6. Coffee

The sirtfood diet gives you another good reason to enjoy a good cup of coffee in the morning, that's right! Coffee is also rich in sirtuins. Along with that, it can give you boosting energy as it can accelerate metabolism.

7. Turmeric

Turmeric is another super sirtfood that is often used in treatments due to its anti-inflammatory, antiseptic, and antioxidant properties. Turmeric contains a compound known as curcumin, which gives this spice a bright color and also protects against the threats of certain cancers, Alzheimer's, and blood clots.

Other Sirtuin-Rich Food

There are several other food items that are considered rich in sirtuins. They can be added to daily meals to increase your sirtuins intake. Enjoy the mix of these ingredients to have a variety of flavor on your platter.

- ➢ Buckwheat
- ➢ Capers
- ➢ Parsley
- ➢ Celery
- ➢ Chili
- ➢ Kale
- ➢ Lovage
- ➢ Extra virgin olive oil
- ➢ Medjool dates
- ➢ Red chicory
- ➢ Rocket
- ➢ Soy
- ➢ Strawberries
- ➢ Walnuts

Sirtfood Diet Phases

For every newbie, it is important to understand that the sirtfood diet does not start with a single list of ingredients in your hands. Its implementation and adaptation are more than mere selective grocery shopping. Every diet can only work effectively when we allow our body to embrace the sudden shift and change in food intake. Similarly, the sirtfood diet also comes with two phases of adaptation. If a dieter successfully goes through these phases, he can continue with the sirtfood diet easily. There are mainly two phases of this diet which are then succeeded by a third phase in which you can decide how you want to continue the diet.

Phase One

The first seven days of this diet plan are characterized as Phase One. In this phase, a dieter must focus on calorie restriction and the intake of green juices. These seven days are crucial to initiate your weight loss and usually helps to lose up to seven pounds if the diet is followed properly. If you find yourself achieving this target, that means that you are on the right track.

In the first three days of the first phase, a dieter must restrict this caloric intake to 1,000 calories only. While doing so, the dieter must also have green juice throughout the day, probably three times a day. Try to drink green juice per meal. The recipes given in the book are perfect to select from. Pick a recipe given in their respective chapters and pair each with green juices.

There are many meal options that can keep your caloric intake in check such as buckwheat noodles, seared tofu, some shrimp stir fry, or sirtfood omelet.

Once the first three days of this diet has passed, you can increase your caloric intake to 1,500 calories per day. In these next four days, you can reduce the green juices to two times per side. And pair the juices with more Sirtuin-rich food in every meal.

Phase Two

After the first week of the sirtfood diet, then starts phase two. This phase is more about the maintenance of the diet, as the first week enables the body to embrace the change and start working according to the new diet. This phase enables the body to continue working towards the weight loss objective slowly and steadily. Therefore, the duration of this phase is almost two weeks.

So how is this phase different from the phase one? In this phase, there is no restriction on the caloric intake, as long as the food is rich in sirtuins and you are taking it three times a day, it is good to go. Instead of having the green juice two or three times a day, the dieter can have juice one time a day, and that will be enough to achieve steady weight loss. You can have the juice after any meal, in the morning or in the evening.

After the Diet Phase

With the end of phase two comes the time which is most crucial, and that is the after-diet phase. If you haven't achieved your weight loss target by the end of phase two, then you can restart the phases all over again. Or even when you have achieved the goals but still want to lose more weight, then you can again give it a try.

Instead of following phases one and two over and over again, you can also continue having good quality sirtfood meals in this after-diet phase. Simply continue the eating practices of phase two, have a diet rich in sirtuin, and do have green juices whenever possible.

PHASE 1 RECIPES

Matcha Green Juice

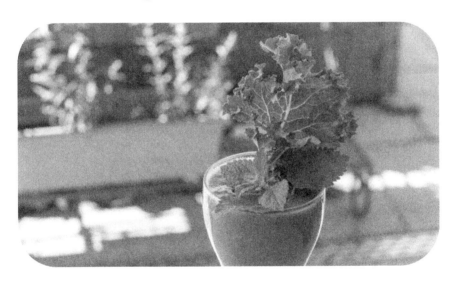

Ingredients

- ➤ 5 ounces fresh kale
- ➤ 2 ounces fresh arugula
- ➤ ¼ cup fresh parsley
- ➤ 4 celery stalks

- 1 green apple, cored and chopped
- 1 (1-inch) piece fresh ginger, peeled
- 1 lemon, peeled
- ½ teaspoon matcha green tea

How to Prepare

1. Add all ingredients into a juicer and extract the juice according to the manufacturer's method.
2. Pour into 2 glasses and serve immediately.

Preparation time: 10 minutes
Total time: 10 minutes
Servings: 2

Nutritional Values

- Calories 113
- Total Fat 0.6 g
- Saturated Fat 0.1 g
- Cholesterol 0 mg
- Sodium 71 mg
- Total Carbs 26.71 g
- Fiber 5.3 g
- Sugar 12.9 g
- Protein 3.8 g

Celery Juice

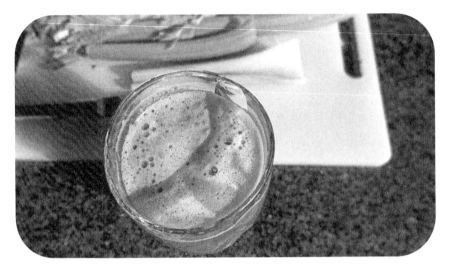

Ingredients

- 8 celery stalks with leaves
- 2 tablespoons fresh ginger, peeled
- 1 lemon, peeled
- ½ cup filtered water
- Pinch of salt

How to Prepare

1. Place all the ingredients in a blender and pulse until well combined.
2. Through a fine mesh strainer, strain the juice and transfer into 2 glasses.

3. Serve immediately.

Preparation time: 10 minutes
Total time: 10 minutes
Servings: 2

Nutritional Values

> ➤ *Calories 32*
> ➤ *Total Fat 0.5 g*
> ➤ *Saturated Fat 0.1 g*
> ➤ *Cholesterol 0 mg*
> ➤ *Sodium 134 mg*
> ➤ *Total Carbs 6.5 g*
> ➤ *Fiber 2 g*
> ➤ *Sugar 1.3 g*
> ➤ *Protein 1 g*

Kale & Orange Juice

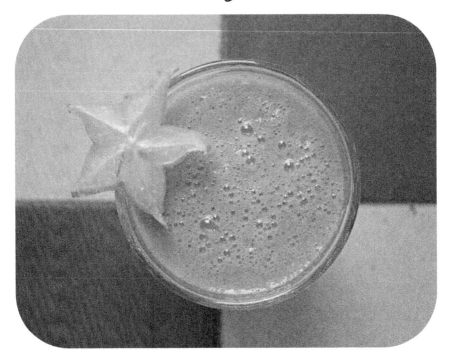

Ingredients

➢ *5 large oranges, peeled and sectioned*

➢ *2 bunches fresh kale*

How to Prepare

1. Add all ingredients into a juicer and extract the juice according to the manufacturer's method.

2. Pour into 2 glasses and serve immediately.

Preparation time: 10 minutes

Total time: 10 minutes

Servings: 2

Nutritional Values

- ➢ *Calories 315*
- ➢ *Total Fat 0.6 g*
- ➢ *Saturated Fat 0.1 g*
- ➢ *Cholesterol 0 mg*
- ➢ *Sodium 87 mg*
- ➢ *Total Carbs 75.1 g*
- ➢ *Fiber 14 g*
- ➢ *Sugar 4.3 g*
- ➢ *Protein 10.3 g*

Apple & Cucumber Juice

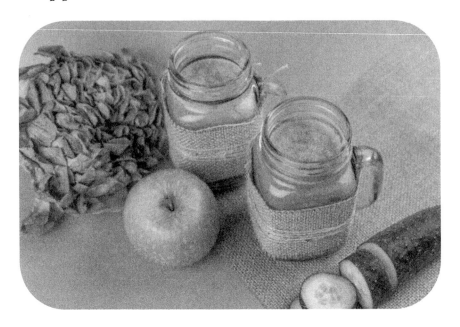

Ingredients

- 3 large apples, cored and sliced
- 2 large cucumbers, sliced
- 4 celery stalks
- 1 (1-inch) piece fresh ginger, peeled
- 1 lemon, peeled

How to Prepare

1. Add all ingredients into a juicer and extract the juice according to the manufacturer's method.
2. Pour into 2 glasses and serve immediately.

Preparation time: 10 minutes

Total time: 10 minutes

Servings: 2

Nutritional Values

- ➤ *Calories 230*
- ➤ *Total Fat 1.1 g*
- ➤ *Saturated Fat 0.1 g*
- ➤ *Cholesterol 0 mg*
- ➤ *Sodium 37 mg*
- ➤ *Total Carbs 59.5 g*
- ➤ *Fiber 10.5 g*
- ➤ *Sugar 40.5 g*
- ➤ *Protein 3.3 g*

Lemony Green Juice

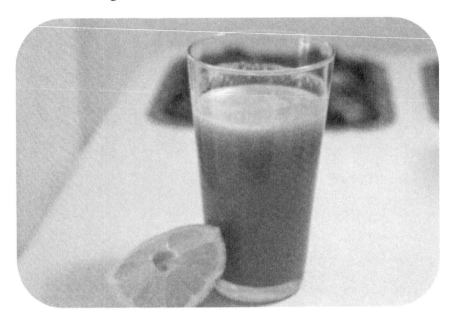

Ingredients

- 2 large green apples, cored and sliced
- 4 cups fresh kale leaves
- 4 tablespoons fresh parsley leaves
- 1 tablespoon fresh ginger, peeled
- 1 lemon, peeled
- ½ cup filtered water
- Pinch of salt

How to Prepare

1. Place all the ingredients in a blender and pulse until well combined.

2. Through a fine mesh strainer, strain the juice and transfer into 2 glasses.

3. Serve immediately.

Preparation time: 10 minutes
Total time: 10 minutes
Servings: 2

Nutritional Values

➢ *Calories 196*
➢ *Total Fat 0.6 g*
➢ *Saturated Fat 0.1 g*
➢ *Cholesterol 0 mg*
➢ *Sodium 143 mg*
➢ *Total Carbs 47.9 g*
➢ *Fiber 8.2 g*
➢ *Sugar 23.5 g*
➢ *Protein 5.2 g*

Kale Scramble

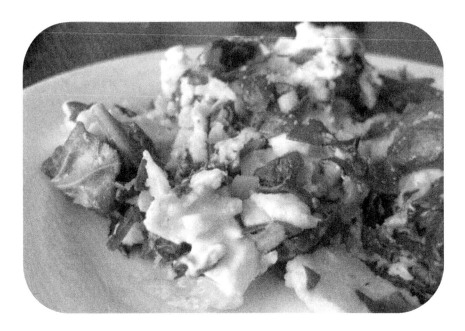

Ingredients

- 4 eggs
- 1/8 teaspoon ground turmeric
- Salt and ground black pepper, to taste
- 1 tablespoon water
- 2 teaspoons olive oil
- 1 cup fresh kale, tough ribs removed and chopped

How to Prepare

1. In a bowl, add the eggs, turmeric, salt, black pepper, and water and with a whisk, beat until foamy.

2. In a wok, heat the oil over medium heat.

3. Add the egg mixture and stir to combine.

4. Immediately, reduce the heat to medium-low and cook for about 1–2 minutes, stirring frequently.

5. Stir in the kale and cook for about 3–4 minutes, stirring frequently.

6. Remove from the heat and serve immediately.

Preparation time: 10 minutes

Cooking time: 6 minutes

Total time: 16 minutes

Servings: 2

Nutritional Values

- *Calories 183*
- *Total Fat 13.4 g*
- *Saturated Fat 3.4 g*
- *Cholesterol 327 mg*
- *Sodium 216 mg*
- *Total Carbs 4.3 g*
- *Fiber 0.5 g*
- *Sugar 0.7 g*
- *Protein 12.1 g*

Buckwheat Porridge

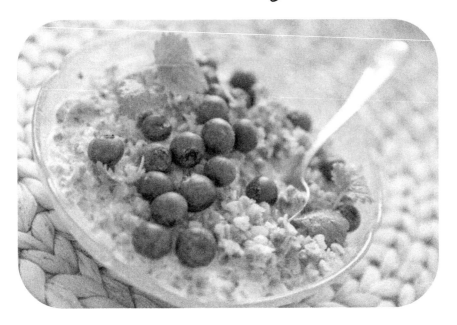

Ingredients

- ➢ 1 cup buckwheat, rinsed
- ➢ 1 cup unsweetened almond milk
- ➢ 1 cup water
- ➢ ½ teaspoon ground cinnamon
- ➢ ½ teaspoon vanilla extract
- ➢ 1–2 tablespoons raw honey
- ➢ ¼ cup fresh blueberries

How to Prepare

1. In a pan, add all the ingredients (except honey and blueberries) over medium-high heat and bring to a boil.

2. Now, reduce the heat to low and simmer, covered for about 10 minutes.

3. Stir in the honey and remove from the heat.

4. Set aside, covered, for about 5 minutes.

5. With a fork, fluff the mixture, and transfer into serving bowls.

6. Top with blueberries and serve.

Preparation time: 10 minutes
Cooking time: 15 minutes
Total time: 25 minutes
Servings: 2

Nutritional Values

➢ *Calories 358*
➢ *Total Fat 4.7 g*
➢ *Saturated Fat 0.8 g*
➢ *Cholesterol 0 mg*
➢ *Sodium 95 mg*
➢ *Total Carbs 3.7 g*
➢ *Fiber 9.8 g*
➢ *Sugar 10.6 g*
➢ *Protein 12 g*

Chocolate Granola

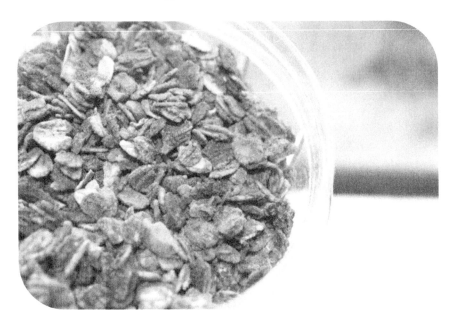

Ingredients

- ¼ cup cacao powder
- ¼ cup maple syrup
- 2 tablespoons coconut oil, melted
- ½ teaspoon vanilla extract
- 1/8 teaspoon salt
- 2 cups gluten-free rolled oats
- ¼ cup unsweetened coconut flakes
- 2 tablespoons chia seeds
- 2 tablespoons unsweetened dark chocolate, chopped finely

How to Prepare

1. Preheat your oven to 300°F and line a medium baking sheet with parchment paper.

2. In a medium pan, add the cacao powder, maple syrup, coconut oil, vanilla extract, and salt, and mix well.

3. Now, place pan over medium heat and cook for about 2–3 minutes, or until thick and syrupy, stirring continuously.

4. Remove from the heat and set aside.

5. In a large bowl, add the oats, coconut, and chia seeds, and mix well.

6. Add the syrup mixture and mix until well combined.

7. Transfer the granola mixture onto a prepared baking sheet and spread in an even layer.

8. Bake for about 35 minutes.

9. Remove from the oven and set aside for about 1 hour.

10. Add the chocolate pieces and stir to combine.

11. Serve immediately.

Preparation time: 10 minutes
Cooking time: 38 minutes
Total time: 48 minutes
Servings: 8

Nutritional Values

➢ *Calories 193*

- ➤ *Total Fat 9.1 g*
- ➤ *Saturated Fat 5.2 g*
- ➤ *Cholesterol 0 mg*
- ➤ *Sodium 37 mg*
- ➤ *Total Carbs 26.1 g*
- ➤ *Fiber 4.6 g*
- ➤ *Sugar 5.9 g*
- ➤ *Protein 5 g*

Blueberry Muffins

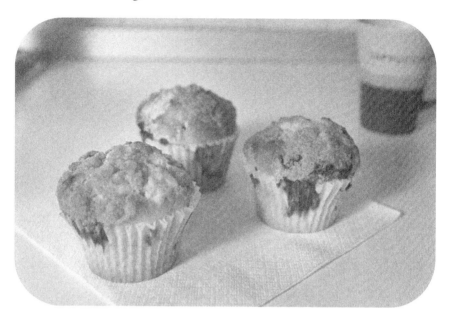

Ingredients

- 1 cup buckwheat flour
- ¼ cup arrowroot starch
- 1½ teaspoons baking powder
- ¼ teaspoon sea salt
- 2 eggs
- ½ cup unsweetened almond milk
- 2–3 tablespoons maple syrup
- 2 tablespoons coconut oil, melted
- 1 cup fresh blueberries

How to Prepare

1. Preheat your oven to 350°F and line 8 cups of a muffin tin.
2. In a bowl, place the buckwheat flour, arrowroot starch, baking powder, and salt, and mix well.
3. In a separate bowl, place the eggs, almond milk, maple syrup, and coconut oil, and beat until well combined.
4. Now, place the flour mixture and mix until just combined.
5. Gently, fold in the blueberries.
6. Transfer the mixture into prepared muffin cups evenly.
7. Bake for about 25 minutes or until a toothpick inserted in the center comes out clean.
8. Remove the muffin tin from oven and place onto a wire rack to cool for about 10 minutes.
9. Carefully invert the muffins onto the wire rack to cool completely before serving.

Preparation time: 15 minutes
Cooking time: 20 minutes
Total time: 35 minutes
Servings: 8

Nutritional Values

- Calories 136
- Total Fat 5.3 g
- Saturated Fat 3.4 g
- Cholesterol 41 mg
- Sodium 88 mg
- Total Carbs 20.7 g
- Fiber 2.2 g
- Sugar 5.7 g
- Protein 3.5 g

Chocolate Waffles

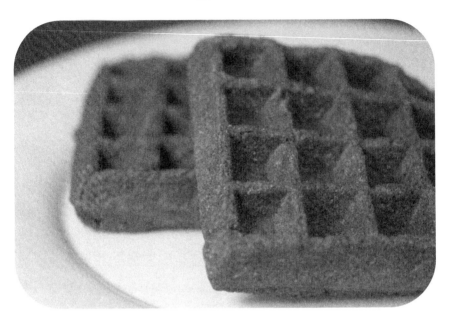

Ingredients

- ➢ 2 cups unsweetened almond milk
- ➢ 1 tablespoon fresh lemon juice
- ➢ 1 cup buckwheat flour
- ➢ ½ cup cacao powder
- ➢ ¼ cup flaxseed meal
- ➢ 1 teaspoon baking soda
- ➢ 1 teaspoon baking powder
- ➢ ¼ teaspoons kosher salt
- ➢ 2 large eggs
- ➢ ½ cup coconut oil, melted

- ➢ ¼ cup dark brown sugar
- ➢ 2 teaspoons vanilla extract
- ➢ 2 ounces unsweetened dark chocolate, chopped roughly

How to Prepare

1. In a bowl, add the almond milk and lemon juice and mix well.
2. Set aside for about 10 minutes.
3. In a bowl, place buckwheat flour, cacao powder, flaxseed meal, baking soda, baking powder, and salt, and mix well.
4. In the bowl of almond milk mixture, place the eggs, coconut oil, brown sugar, and vanilla extract, and beat until smooth.
5. Now, place the flour mixture and beat until smooth.
6. Gently, fold in the chocolate pieces.
7. Preheat the waffle iron and then grease it.
8. Place the desired amount of the mixture into the preheated waffle iron and cook for about 3 minutes, or until golden-brown.
9. Repeat with the remaining mixture.

Preparation time: 15 minutes
Cooking time: 24 minutes
Total time: 39 minutes
Servings: 8

Nutritional Values

- Calories 295
- Total Fat 22.1 g
- Saturated Fat 15.5 g
- Cholesterol 47 mg
- Sodium 302 mg
- Total Carbs 1.5 g
- Fiber 5.2 g
- Sugar 5.1 g
- Protein 6.3 g

Salmon & Kale Omelet

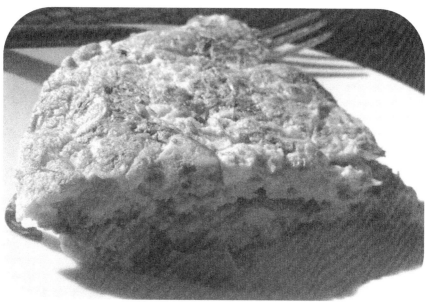

Ingredients

- 6 eggs
- 2 tablespoons unsweetened almond milk
- Salt and ground black pepper, to taste
- 2 tablespoons olive oil
- 4 ounces smoked salmon, cut into bite-sized chunks
- 2 cup fresh kale, tough ribs removed and chopped finely
- 4 scallions, chopped finely

How to Prepare

1. In a bowl, place the eggs, coconut milk, salt, and black pepper, and beat well. Set aside.
2. In a non-stick wok, heat the oil over medium heat.

3. Place the egg mixture evenly and cook for about 30 seconds, without stirring.
4. Place the salmon kale and scallions on top of egg mixture evenly.
5. Now, reduce heat to low.
6. With the lid, cover the wok and cook for about 4–5 minutes, or until omelet is done completely.
7. Uncover the wok and cook for about 1 minute.
8. Carefully, transfer the omelet onto a serving plate and serve.

Preparation time: 10 minutes
Cooking time: 7 minutes
Total time: 17 minutes
Servings: 4

Nutritional Values

➢ *Calories 210*
➢ *Total Fat 14.9 g*
➢ *Saturated Fat 3.3 g*
➢ *Cholesterol 252 mg*
➢ *Sodium 682 mg*
➢ *Total Carbs 5.2 g*
➢ *Fiber 0.9 g*
➢ *Sugar 0.9 g*
➢ *Protein 14.8 g*

Eggs with Kale

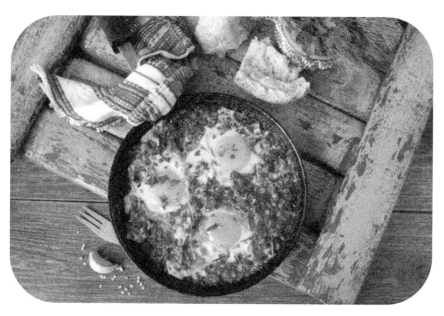

Ingredients

- ➢ 2 tablespoons olive oil
- ➢ 1 yellow onion, chopped
- ➢ 2 garlic cloves, minced
- ➢ 1 cup tomatoes, chopped
- ➢ ½ pound fresh kale, tough ribs removed and chopped
- ➢ 1 teaspoon ground cumin
- ➢ ¼ teaspoon red pepper flakes, crushed
- ➢ Salt and ground black pepper, to taste
- ➢ 4 eggs
- ➢ 2 tablespoons fresh parsley, chopped

How to Prepare

1. Heat the oil in a large wok over medium heat and sauté the onion for about 4–5 minutes.
2. Add garlic and sauté for about 1 minute.
3. Add the tomatoes, spices, salt, and black pepper, and cook for about 2–3 minutes, stirring frequently.
4. Stir in the kale and cook for about 4–5 minutes.
5. Carefully, crack eggs on top of kale mixture.
6. With the lid, cover the wok and cook for about 10 minutes, or until desired doneness of eggs.
7. Serve hot with the garnishing of parsley.

Preparation time: 15 minutes
Cooking time: 25 minutes
Total time: 40 minutes
Servings: 4

Nutritional Values

- *Calories 175*
- *Total Fat 11.7 g*
- *Saturated Fat 2.4 g*
- *Cholesterol 164 mg*
- *Sodium 130 mg*
- *Total Carbs 11.5 g*
- *Fiber 2.2 g*
- *Sugar 2.8 g*
- *Protein 8.2 g*

Kale & Raspberry Salad

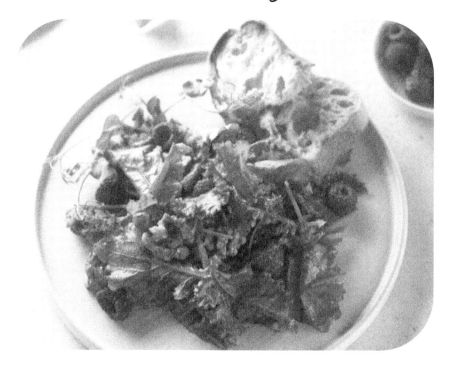

Ingredients

Salad

- 3 cups fresh baby kale
- ½ cup fresh raspberries
- ¼ cup walnuts, chopped

Dressing

- 1 tablespoon extra-virgin olive oil
- 1 tablespoon apple cider vinegar

- ½ teaspoon pure maple syrup
- Salt and ground black pepper, to taste

How to Prepare

1. For salad: in a salad bowl, place all ingredients and mix.
2. For dressing: place all ingredients in another bowl and beat until well combined.
3. Place dressing on top of salad and toss to coat well.
4. Serve immediately.

Preparation time: 15 minutes
Total time: 15 minutes
Servings: 2

Nutritional Values

- *Calories 228*
- *Total Fat 16.4 g*
- *Saturated Fat 1.5 g*
- *Cholesterol 0 mg*
- *Sodium 122 mg*
- *Total Carbs 16.9 g*
- *Fiber 4.6 g*
- *Sugar 2.6 g*
- *Protein 7.1 g*

Kale & Citrus Fruit Salad

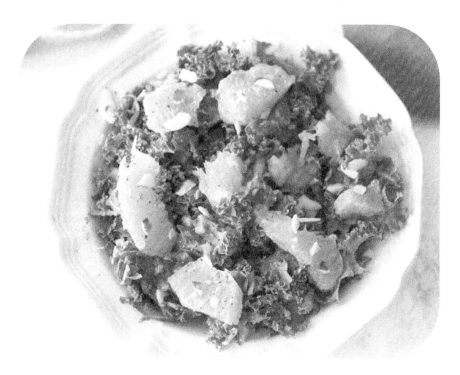

Ingredients

Salad
- 3 cups fresh kale, tough ribs removed and torn
- 1 orange, peeled and segmented
- 1 grapefruit, peeled and segmented
- 2 tablespoons unsweetened dried cranberries
- ¼ teaspoon white sesame seeds

Dressing
- 2 tablespoons extra-virgin olive oil

- ➢ 2 tablespoons fresh orange juice
- ➢ 1 teaspoon Dijon mustard
- ➢ ½ teaspoon raw honey
- ➢ Salt and ground black pepper, to taste

How to Prepare

1. For salad: in a salad bowl, place all ingredients and mix.
2. For dressing: place all ingredients in another bowl and beat until well combined.
3. Place dressing on top of salad and toss to coat well.
4. Serve immediately.

Preparation time: 15 minutes

Total time: 15 minutes

Servings: 2

Nutritional Values

- ➢ *Calories 256*
- ➢ *Total Fat 14.5g*
- ➢ *Saturated Fat 2.1 g*
- ➢ *Cholesterol 0 mg*
- ➢ *Sodium 150 mg*
- ➢ *Total Carbs 31.3 g*
- ➢ *Fiber 4.8 g*
- ➢ *Sugar 16.6 g*
- ➢ *Protein 4.6 g*

Arugula & Berries Salad

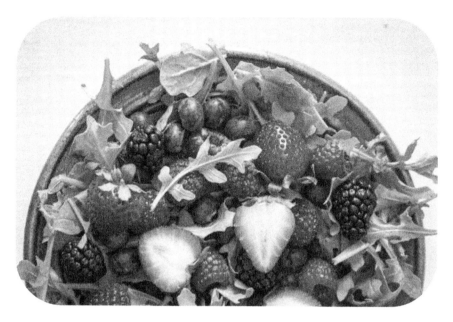

Ingredients
- 1 cup fresh strawberries, hulled and sliced
- ½ cup fresh blackberries
- ½ cup fresh blueberries
- ½ cup fresh raspberries
- 6 cups fresh arugula
- 2 tablespoons extra-virgin olive oil
- Salt and ground black pepper, to taste

How to Prepare
1. In a salad bowl, place all the ingredients and toss to coat well.

2. Serve immediately.

Preparation time: 15 minutes
Total time: 15 minutes
Servings: 4

Nutritional Values

- ➤ *Calories 105*
- ➤ *Total Fat 7.6 g*
- ➤ *Saturated Fat 1 g*
- ➤ *Cholesterol 0 mg*
- ➤ *Sodium 48 mg*
- ➤ *Total Carbs 10.1 g*
- ➤ *Fiber 3.6 g*
- ➤ *Sugar 5.7 g*
- ➤ *Protein 1.6 g*

Rocket & Orange Salad

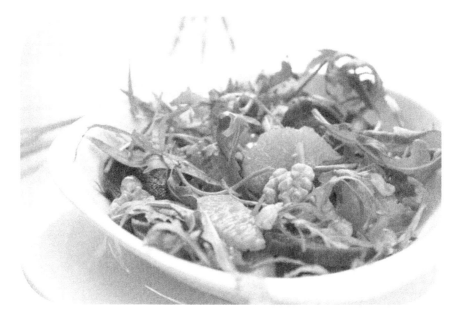

Ingredients

- 3 large oranges, peeled, seeded, and sectioned
- 2 beets, trimmed, peeled, and sliced
- 6 cups fresh rocket
- ¼ cup walnuts, chopped
- 3 tablespoons olive oil
- Pinch of salt

How to Prepare

1. In a salad bowl, place all ingredients and gently, toss to coat.

2. Serve immediately.

Preparation time: 10 minutes
Total time: 10 minutes
Servings: 4

Nutritional Values

➢ *Calories 233*
➢ *Total Fat 15.6 g*
➢ *Saturated Fat 1.8 g*
➢ *Cholesterol 0 mg*
➢ *Sodium 86 mg*
➢ *Total Carbs 23.1 g*
➢ *Fiber 5.3 g*
➢ *Sugar 17.6 g*
➢ *Protein 4.8 g*

Chicken, Kale, & Carrot Salad

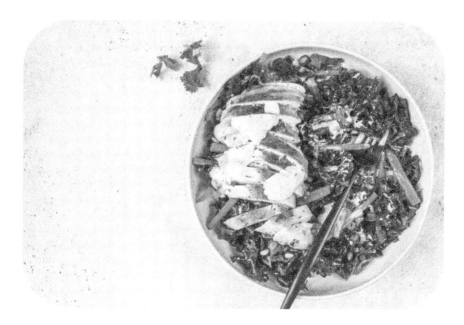

Ingredients

Chicken

- ➢ 1 teaspoon dried thyme
- ➢ ½ teaspoon garlic powder
- ➢ ½ teaspoon onion powder
- ➢ ¼ teaspoon cayenne pepper
- ➢ ¼ teaspoon ground turmeric
- ➢ Salt and ground black pepper, to taste

- ➢ 2 (7-ounce) boneless, skinless chicken breasts, pounded into ¾-inch thickness
- ➢ 1 tablespoon olive oil

Salad
- ➢ 5 cups fresh kale, tough ribs removed and chopped
- ➢ 1½ cups carrots, peeled and cut into matchsticks
- ➢ ¼ cup pine nuts

Dressing
- ➢ 1 small garlic clove, minced
- ➢ 2 tablespoons fresh lime juice
- ➢ 2 tablespoons extra-virgin olive oil
- ➢ 1 teaspoon raw honey
- ➢ ½ teaspoon Dijon mustard
- ➢ Salt and ground black pepper, to taste

How to Prepare

1. Preheat your oven to 425°F and line a baking dish with parchment paper.
2. For chicken: in a bowl, mix together the thyme, spices, salt, and black pepper.
3. Drizzle the chicken breasts with oil and then rub with spice mixture generously and drizzle with the oil.
4. Arrange the chicken breasts onto the prepared baking dish.

5. Bake for about 16–18 minutes.
6. Remove pan from oven, transfer chicken breasts onto a cutting board for about 5 minutes.
7. For salad: place all ingredients in a salad bowl and mix.
8. For dressing: place all ingredients in another bowl and beat until well combined.
9. Cut each chicken breast into desired sized slices.
10. Place the salad onto each serving plate and top each with chicken slices.
11. Drizzle with dressing and serve.

Preparation time: 15 minutes
Cooking time: 18 minutes
Total time: 33 minutes
Servings: 4

Nutritional Values

➢ *Calories 330*
➢ *Total Fat 18.9 g*
➢ *Saturated Fat 1.9 g*
➢ *Cholesterol 64 mg*
➢ *Sodium 162 mg*
➢ *Total Carbs 16.5 g*
➢ *Fiber 2.8 g*
➢ *Sugar 4 g*
➢ *Protein 25.3 g*

Veggie Burgers

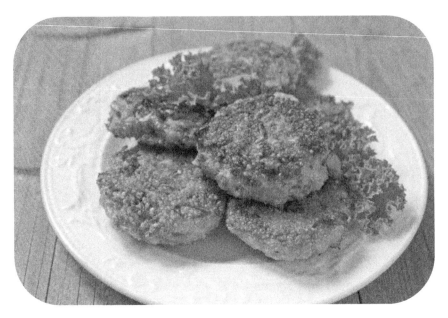

Ingredients

- ➢ 1 cup water
- ➢ 1/3 cup dry couscous
- ➢ 1½ cups broccoli florets
- ➢ 2 teaspoons olive oil
- ➢ ½ cup onion, chopped
- ➢ ½ cup scallion, chopped
- ➢ 2 teaspoons ground cumin
- ➢ ¼ teaspoon ground turmeric
- ➢ 1 tablespoon sesame tahini
- ➢ 1 (15-ounce) can chickpeas, rinsed and drained

- ½ cup panko breadcrumbs
- 4 cups fresh kale, tough ribs removed and chopped

How to Prepare

1. Preheat your oven to 400°F. Line a baking sheet with foil paper.
2. In a small pan, mix together water and couscous over medium heat and bring to a boil.
3. Immediately, remove from heat and set aside, covered for about 10 minutes, or until all the liquid is absorbed.
4. Meanwhile, in a pan of boiling water, arrange a steamer basket.
5. Place the broccoli in steamer basket and steam, covered for about 5–7 minutes.
6. Drain the broccoli well.
7. Meanwhile, in a wok, heat the oil over medium heat and sauté the onion and scallion for about 3–5 minutes.
8. Stir in the cumin and turmeric and remove from heat.
9. In a food processor, add the couscous, broccoli, onion mixture, tahini, and chickpeas, and pulse until well combined.
10. Transfer the mixture into a bowl.
11. Add the breadcrumbs and stir to combine.
12. Make equal-sized patties from mixture.

13. Arrange the patties onto the prepared baking sheet in a single layer.

14. Bake for about 50 minutes, flipping once halfway through.

15. Divide kale among 4 serving plates.

16. Top each plate with 1 patty and serve.

Preparation time: 20 minutes

Cooking time: 10 minutes

Total time: 30 minutes

Servings: 4

Nutritional Values

➢ *Calories 321*

➢ *Total Fat 7.1 g*

➢ *Saturated Fat 1.1 g*

➢ *Cholesterol 0 mg*

➢ *Sodium 76 mg*

➢ *Total Carbs 44.2 g*

➢ *Fiber 8.3 g*

➢ *Sugar 1.5 g*

➢ *Protein 12.8 g*

Kale with Pine Nuts

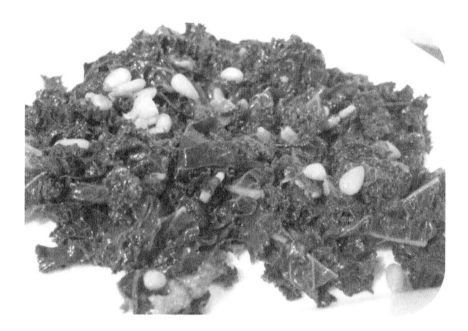

Ingredients

- ➤ 1 tablespoon olive oil
- ➤ 2 garlic cloves, minced
- ➤ 1½ pounds fresh kale, tough ribs removed and chopped
- ➤ ¼ cup water
- ➤ 3 teaspoons red wine vinegar
- ➤ Salt and ground black pepper, to taste
- ➤ 2 tablespoons pine nuts

How to Prepare

1. Heat the olive oil in a large wok over medium heat and sauté the garlic for about 1 minute.

2. Add kale and cook for about 3–4 minutes.
3. Add the water, vinegar, salt, and black pepper, and cook for 4–5 minutes.
4. Remove from heat and stir in the pine nuts.
5. Serve immediately.

Preparation time: 10 minutes
Cooking time: 10 minutes
Total time: 20 minutes
Servings: 4

Nutritional Values

- *Calories 146*
- *Total Fat 6.5 g*
- *Saturated Fat 0.7 g*
- *Cholesterol 0 mg*
- *Sodium 113 mg*
- *Total Carbs 18.9 g*
- *Fiber 2.7 g*
- *Sugar 0.2 g*
- *Protein 5.8 g*

Bok Choy & Mushroom Stir Fry

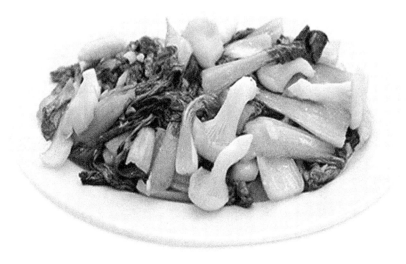

Ingredients

- ➢ 1 pound baby bok choy
- ➢ 4 teaspoons olive oil
- ➢ 1 teaspoon fresh ginger, minced
- ➢ 2 garlic cloves, chopped
- ➢ 5 ounces fresh mushrooms, sliced
- ➢ 2 tablespoons red wine
- ➢ 2 tablespoons soy sauce
- ➢ Ground black pepper, to taste

How to Prepare

1. Trim bases of bok choy and separate outer leaves from stalks, leaving the smallest inner leaves attached.
2. In a large cast-iron wok, heat the oil over medium-high heat and sauté the ginger and garlic for about 1 minute.
3. Stir in the mushrooms and cook for about 4–5 minutes, stirring frequently.
4. Stir in the bok choy leaves and stalks and cook for about 1 minute, tossing with tongs.
5. Stir in the wine, soy sauce, and black pepper, and cook for about 2–3 minutes, tossing occasionally.
6. Serve hot.

Preparation time: 15 minutes
Cooking time: 10 minutes
Total time: 25 minutes
Servings: 4

Nutritional Values

- *Calories 77*
- *Total Fat 5 g*
- *Saturated Fat 0.7 g*
- *Cholesterol 0 mg*
- *Sodium 527 mg*
- *Total Carbs 5.3 g*
- *Fiber 1.6 g*
- *Sugar 2.2 g*
- *Protein 3.5 g*

Shrimp with Kale

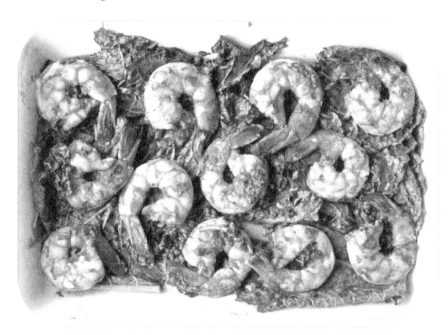

Ingredients

- 3 tablespoons olive oil
- 1 pound medium shrimp, peeled and deveined
- 1 medium onion, chopped
- 4 garlic cloves, chopped finely
- 1 fresh red chili, sliced
- 1 pound fresh kale, tough ribs removed and chopped
- ¼ cup low-sodium chicken broth

How to Prepare

1. In a large non-stick wok, heat 1 tablespoon of the oil over medium-high heat and cook the shrimp for about 2 minutes per side.

2. With a slotted spoon, transfer the shrimp onto a plate.

3. In the same wok, heat the remaining 2 tablespoons of oil over medium heat and sauté the garlic and red chili for about 1 minute.

4. Add the kale and broth and cook for about 4–5 minutes, stirring occasionally.

5. Stir in the cooked shrimp and cook for about 1 minute.

6. Serve hot.

Preparation time: 15 minutes
Cooking time: 10 minutes
Total time: 25 minutes
Servings: 4

Nutritional Values

➢ *Calories 270*
➢ *Total Fat 11.9 g*
➢ *Saturated Fat 1.5 g*
➢ *Cholesterol 223 mg*
➢ *Sodium 312 mg*
➢ *Total Carbs 15.5 g*
➢ *Fiber 2.3 g*
➢ *Sugar 1.2 g*
➢ *Protein 28.3 g*

Prawns with Asparagus

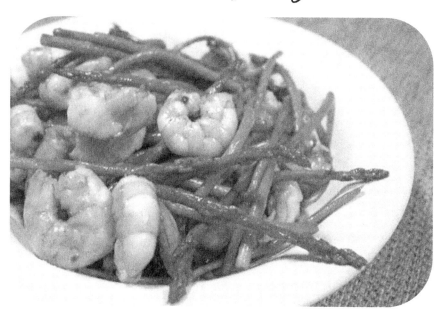

Ingredients

- 3 tablespoons olive oil
- 1 pound prawns, peeled, and deveined
- 1 pound asparagus, trimmed
- Salt and ground black pepper, to taste
- 1 teaspoon garlic, minced
- 1 teaspoon fresh ginger, minced
- 1 tablespoon low-sodium soy sauce
- 2 tablespoons lemon juice

How to Prepare

1. In a wok, heat 2 tablespoons of oil over medium-high heat and cook the prawns with salt and black pepper for about 3–4 minutes.

2. With a slotted spoon, transfer the prawns into a bowl. Set aside.
3. In the same wok, heat remaining 1 tablespoon of oil over medium-high heat and cook the asparagus, ginger, garlic, salt, and black pepper and sauté for about 6–8 minutes, stirring frequently.
4. Stir in the prawns and soy sauce and cook for about 1 minute.
5. Stir in the lemon juice and remove from the heat.
6. Serve hot.

Preparation time: 15 minutes
Cooking time: 13 minutes
Total time: 28 minutes
Servings: 4

Nutritional Values

➢ *Calories 253*
➢ *Total Fat 12.7 g*
➢ *Saturated Fat 2.2 g*
➢ *Cholesterol 239 mg*
➢ *Sodium 501 mg*
➢ *Total Carbs 7.1 g*
➢ *Fiber 2.5 g*
➢ *Sugar 2.6 g*
➢ *Protein 28.7 g*

Kale with Tofu & Chickpeas

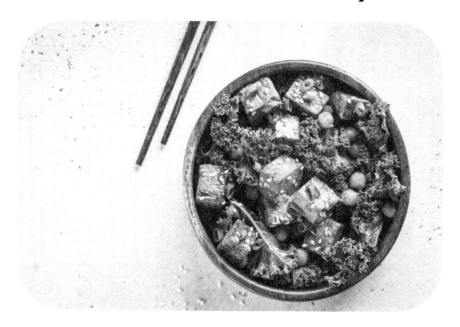

Ingredients

Tofu

- ➤ 2 tablespoons olive oil
- ➤ 12 ounces tofu, drained, pressed, and cut into 1-inch cubes
- ➤ 1 tablespoon soy sauce
- ➤ 1 teaspoon maple syrup
- ➤ 1 tablespoon red pepper flakes
- ➤ ¼ cup water

Chickpeas & Kale

- 2 tablespoons olive oil
- 1½ (14-ounce) cans chickpeas, rinsed and drained
- ¼ teaspoon ground turmeric
- Salt and ground black pepper, to taste
- 6 cups fresh baby kale
- 1 teaspoon sesame seeds

How to Prepare

1. For tofu: in a large cast-iron wok, heat the olive oil over medium heat and cook the tofu cubes for about 8–10 minutes, or until golden from all sides.
2. Add the remaining ingredients and cook for about 2-3 minutes.
3. Meanwhile, for chickpeas mixture: in another wok, heat the oil over medium heat and cook the chickpeas, turmeric, salt, and black pepper for about 2–3 minutes.
4. Remove from the transfer the chickpeas into a large bowl.
5. Add the tofu mixture and kale and stir to combine.
6. Garnish with sesame seeds and serve.

Preparation time: 20 minutes
Cooking time: 15 minutes
Total time: 35 minutes
Servings: 4

Nutritional Values

- Calories 370
- Total Fat 20.5 g
- Saturated Fat 2.8 g
- Cholesterol 0 mg
- Sodium 658 mg
- Total Carbs 35 g
- Fiber 9.7 g
- Sugar 2.9 g
- Protein 17.4 g

Lentil & Greens Soup

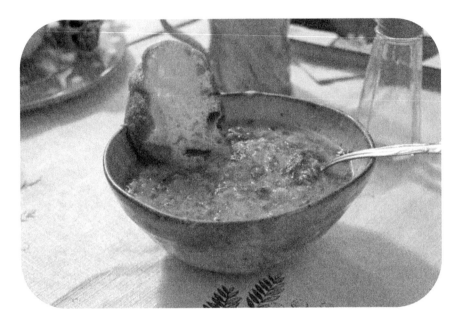

Ingredients

- ➢ 1 tablespoon olive oil
- ➢ 2 carrots, peeled and chopped
- ➢ 2 celery stalks, chopped
- ➢ 1 medium yellow onion, chopped
- ➢ 3 garlic cloves, minced
- ➢ 1½ teaspoon ground cumin
- ➢ 1 teaspoon ground turmeric
- ➢ ¼ teaspoon red pepper flakes
- ➢ 1 (14½-ounce) can diced tomatoes
- ➢ 1 cup red lentils, rinsed

- ➤ 5½ cups water
- ➤ 2 cups fresh mustard greens, chopped
- ➤ Salt and ground black pepper, to taste
- ➤ 2 tablespoons fresh lemon juice

How to Prepare

1. Heat olive oil in a large pan over medium heat and sauté the carrots, celery, and onion for about 5–6 minutes.
2. Add the garlic and spices and sauté for about 1 minute.
3. Add the tomatoes and cook for about 2–3 minutes.
4. Stir in the lentils and water and bring to a boil.
5. Now, reduce the heat to low and simmer, covered for about 35 minutes.
6. Stir in greens and cook for about 5 minutes.
7. Stir in salt, black pepper, and lemon juice, and remove from the heat.
8. Serve hot.

Preparation time: 15 minutes
Cooking time: 55 minutes
Total time: 1 hour 10 minutes
Servings: 6

Nutritional Values

- Calories 174
- Total Fat 3.1 g
- Saturated Fat 0.5 g
- Cholesterol 0 mg
- Sodium 59 mg
- Total Carbs 27.8 g
- Fiber 12.4 g
- Sugar 4.8 g
- Protein 10 g

Buckwheat Noodles with Veggies

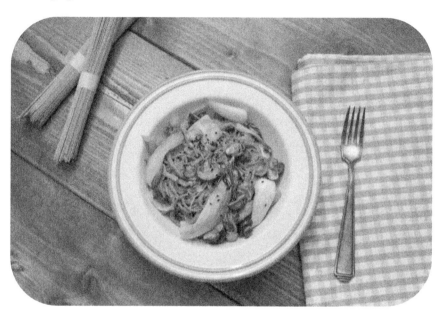

Ingredients

- ➢ 8 ounces buckwheat noodles
- ➢ 2 tablespoons olive oil
- ➢ 1 shallot, minced
- ➢ 1 cup fresh mushrooms, sliced
- ➢ 2 carrots, peeled and sliced diagonally
- ➢ 1½ cups bok choy, chopped
- ➢ 1/3 cup low-sodium vegetable broth
- ➢ 1 tablespoon low-sodium soy sauce

How to Prepare

1. In a pan of lightly salted boiling water, cook the soba noodles for about 5 minutes.

2. Drain the noodles well and rinse under cold water. Set aside.

3. Heat the oil in a large wok over medium-high heat and sauté the shallots for about 3 minutes.

4. Add the mushrooms and stir fry for about 4–5 minutes.

5. Add the carrots and stir fry for about 3 minutes.

6. Add the bok choy and stir fry for about 2–3 minutes.

7. Add the broth and simmer for about 2 minutes.

8. Add the soy sauce and noodles and cook for about 1–2 minutes, tossing occasionally.

9. Serve hot.

Preparation time: 20 minutes
Cooking time: 25 minutes
Total time: 45 minutes
Servings: 4

Nutritional Values

➢ *Calories 275*
➢ *Total Fat 8.9 g*
➢ *Saturated Fat 1.4 g*
➢ *Cholesterol 0 mg*
➢ *Sodium 272 mg*
➢ *Total Carbs 45.3 g*
➢ *Fiber 6.9 g*
➢ *Sugar 3.8 g*
➢ *Protein 8.9 g*

Chocolate Bites

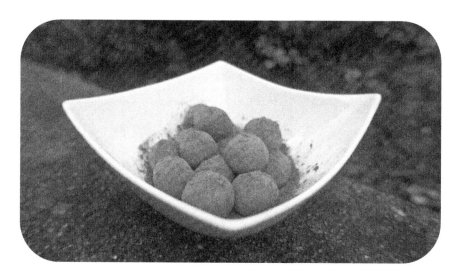

Ingredients

- 1 cup dates, pitted
- 2/3 cup gluten-free rolled oats
- ¼ cup unsweetened dark chocolate, chopped roughly
- 1 tablespoon chia seeds
- 3 tablespoons almond butter
- ½ cup cacao powder

How to Prepare

1. In a food processor, place dates and pulse until finely chopped.

2. Add the remaining ingredients except for cacao powder and pulse until just combined.
3. Make 1-ich balls from the mixture.
4. In a shallow plate, place the cacao powder.
5. Coat the balls with cacao powder and arrange onto a parchment paper-lined baking sheet.
6. Freeze for 15 minutes or until set completely before serving.

Preparation time: 15 minutes
Total time: 15 minutes
Servings: 15

Nutritional Values

➤ *Calories 104*
➤ *Total Fat 5 g*
➤ *Saturated Fat 1.8 g*
➤ *Cholesterol 0 mg*
➤ *Sodium 2 mg*
➤ *Total Carbs 15 g*
➤ *Fiber 3.2 g*
➤ *Sugar 7.7 g*
➤ *Protein 2.8 g*

PHASE 2 RECIPES

Apple & Celery Juice

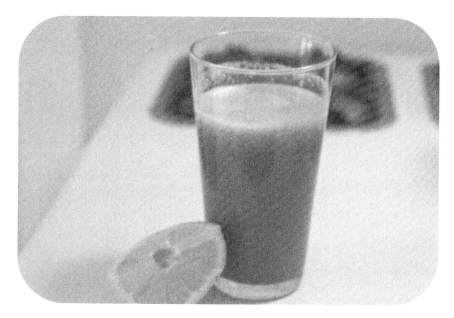

Ingredients

- ➢ 4 large green apples, cored and sliced
- ➢ 4 celery stalks
- ➢ 1 lemon, peeled

How to Prepare

1. Add all ingredients into a juicer and extract the juice according to the manufacturer's method.
2. Pour into 2 glasses and serve immediately.

Preparation time: 10 minutes
Total time: 10 minutes
Servings: 2

Nutritional Values

- Calories 240
- Total Fat 0.9 g
- Saturated Fat 0 g
- Cholesterol 0 mg
- Sodium 31 mg
- Total Carbs 63.3 g
- Fiber 11.6 g
- Sugar 47.1 g
- Protein 1.5 g

Broccoli, Apple, & Orange Juice

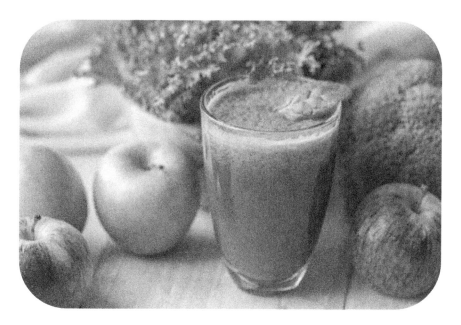

Ingredients

- ➤ 2 broccoli stalks, chopped
- ➤ 2 large green apples, cored and sliced
- ➤ 3 large oranges, peeled and sectioned
- ➤ 4 tablespoons fresh parsley

How to Prepare

1. Add all ingredients into a juicer and extract the juice according to the manufacturer's method.

2. Pour into 2 glasses and serve immediately.

Preparation time: 10 minutes

Total time: 10 minutes

Servings: 2

Nutritional Values

- *Calories 254*
- *Total Fat 0.8 g*
- *Saturated Fat 0.1 g*
- *Cholesterol 0 mg*
- *Sodium 11 mg*
- *Total Carbs 64.7 g*
- *Fiber 12.7 g*
- *Sugar 49.3 g*
- *Protein 3.8 g*

Green Fruit Juice

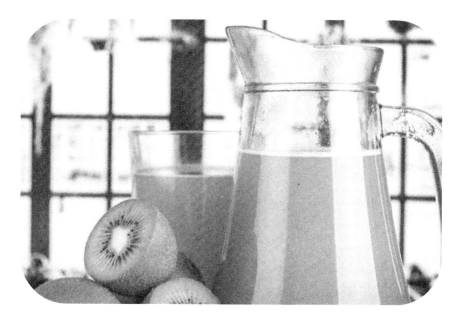

Ingredients

- ➤ 3 large kiwis, peeled and chopped
- ➤ 3 large green apples, cored and sliced
- ➤ 2 cups seedless green grapes
- ➤ 2 teaspoons fresh lime juice

How to Prepare

1. Add all ingredients into a juicer and extract the juice according to the manufacturer's method.
2. Pour into 2 glasses and serve immediately.

Preparation time: 10 minutes

Total time: 10 minutes

Servings: 2

Nutritional Values

- ➢ Calories 304
- ➢ Total Fat 2.2 g
- ➢ Saturated Fat 0 g
- ➢ Cholesterol 0 mg
- ➢ Sodium 6 mg
- ➢ Total Carbs 79 g
- ➢ Fiber 12.5 g
- ➢ Sugar 60.1 g
- ➢ Protein 6.2 g

Kale & Fruit Juice

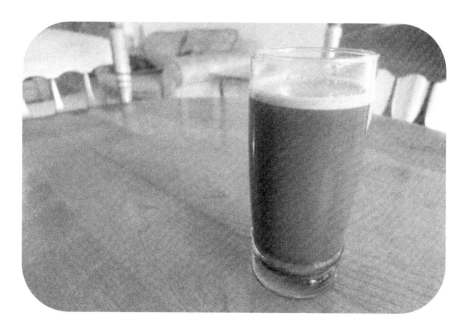

Ingredients

- 2 large green apples, cored and sliced
- 2 large pears, cored and sliced
- 3 cups fresh kale leaves
- 3 celery stalks
- 1 lemon, peeled

How to Prepare

1. Add all ingredients into a juicer and extract the juice according to the manufacturer's method.
2. Pour into 2 glasses and serve immediately.

Preparation time: 10 minutes

Total time: 10 minutes

Servings: 2

Nutritional Values

- ➢ Calories 293
- ➢ Total Fat 0.8 g
- ➢ Saturated Fat 0 g
- ➢ Cholesterol 0 mg
- ➢ Sodium 69 mg
- ➢ Total Carbs 74.6 g
- ➢ Fiber 14 g
- ➢ Sugar 44.1 g
- ➢ Protein 4.6 g

Kale, Carrot, & Grapefruit Juice

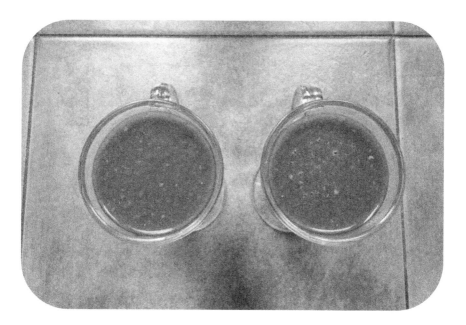

Ingredients

- ➢ 3 cups fresh kale
- ➢ 2 large Granny Smith apples, cored and sliced
- ➢ 2 medium carrots, peeled and chopped
- ➢ 2 medium grapefruit, peeled and sectioned
- ➢ 1 teaspoon fresh lemon juice

How to Prepare

1. Add all ingredients into a juicer and extract the juice according to the manufacturer's method.

2. Pour into 2 glasses and serve immediately.

Preparation time: 10 minutes

Total time: 10 minutes

Servings: 2

Nutritional Values

- ➤ *Calories 232*
- ➤ *Total Fat 0.6 g*
- ➤ *Saturated Fat 0 g*
- ➤ *Cholesterol 0 mg*
- ➤ *Sodium 88 mg*
- ➤ *Total Carbs 57.7 g*
- ➤ *Fiber 9.8 g*
- ➤ *Sugar 35.2 g*
- ➤ *Protein 4.9 g*

Buckwheat Granola

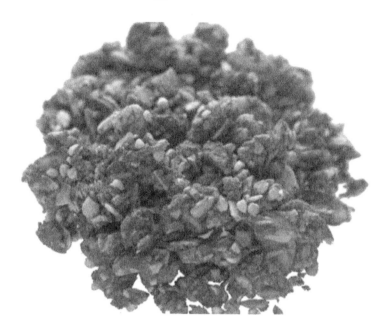

Ingredients

- ➤ 2 cups raw buckwheat groats
- ➤ ¾ cup pumpkin seeds
- ➤ ¾ cup almonds, chopped
- ➤ 1 cup unsweetened coconut flakes
- ➤ 1 teaspoon ground cinnamon
- ➤ 1 teaspoon ground ginger
- ➤ 1 ripe banana, peeled
- ➤ 2 tablespoons maple syrup
- ➤ 2 tablespoons olive oil

How to Prepare

1. Preheat your oven to 350°F.

2. In a bowl, place the buckwheat groats, coconut flakes, pumpkin seeds, almonds, and spices, and mix well.

3. In another bowl, add the banana and with a fork, mash well.

4. Add to the buckwheat mixture maple syrup and oil, and mix until well combined.

5. Transfer the mixture onto the prepared baking sheet and spread in an even layer.

6. Bake for about 25–30 minutes, stirring once halfway through.

7. Remove the baking sheet from oven and set aside to cool.

Preparation time: 15 minutes
Cooking time: 30 minutes
Total time: 45 minutes
Servings: 10

Nutritional Values
➢ *Calories 252*
➢ *Total Fat 14.3 g*
➢ *Saturated Fat 3.7 g*
➢ *Cholesterol 0 mg*
➢ *Sodium 5 mg*
➢ *Total Carbs 27.6 g*
➢ *Fiber 4.9 g*
➢ *Sugar 4.9 g*
➢ *Protein 7.6 g*

Apple Pancakes

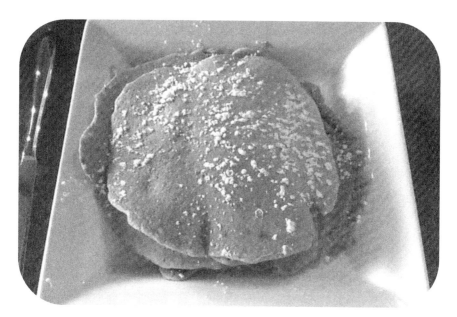

Ingredients

- ½ cup buckwheat flour
- 2 tablespoons coconut sugar
- 1 teaspoon baking powder
- ½ teaspoon ground cinnamon
- 1/3 cup unsweetened almond milk
- 1 egg, beaten lightly
- 2 granny smith apples, peeled, cored, and grated

How to Prepare

1. In a bowl, place the flour, coconut sugar, and cinnamon, and mix well.

2. In another bowl, place the almond milk and egg and beat until well combined.

3. Now, place the flour mixture and mix until well combined.

4. Fold in the grated apples.

5. Heat a lightly greased non-stick wok over medium-high heat.

6. Add desired amount of mixture and with a spoon, spread into an even layer.

7. Cook for 1–2 minutes on each side.

8. Repeat with the remaining mixture.

9. Serve warm with the drizzling of honey.

Preparation time: 15 minutes
Cooking time: 24 minutes
Total time: 39 minutes
Servings: 6

Nutritional Values

- *Calories 93*
- *Total Fat 2.1 g*
- *Saturated Fat 1 g*
- *Cholesterol 27 mg*
- *Sodium 23 mg*
- *Total Carbs 22 g*
- *Fiber 3 g*
- *Sugar 12.1 g*
- *Protein 2.5 g*

Matcha Pancakes

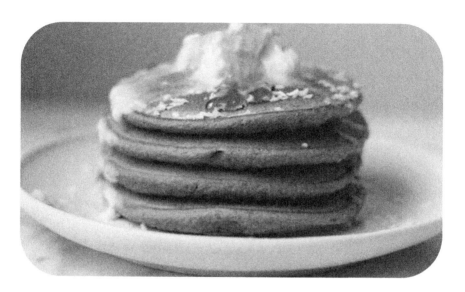

Ingredients

- ➤ 2 tablespoons flax meal
- ➤ 5 tablespoons warm water
- ➤ 1 cup spelt flour
- ➤ 1 cup buckwheat flour
- ➤ 1 tablespoon matcha powder
- ➤ 1 tablespoon baking powder
- ➤ Pinch of salt
- ➤ ¾ cup unsweetened almond milk
- ➤ 1 tablespoon olive oil
- ➤ 1 teaspoon vanilla extract
- ➤ 1/3 cup raw honey

How to Prepare

1. In a bowl, add the flax meal and warm water and mix well. Set aside for about 5 minutes.

2. In another bowl, place the flours, matcha powder, baking powder, and salt, and mix well.

3. In the bowl of flax meal mixture, place the almond milk, oil, and vanilla extract, and beat until well combined.

4. Now, place the flour mixture and mix until a smooth textured mixture is formed.

5. Heat a lightly greased non-stick wok over medium-high heat.

6. Add desired amount of mixture and with a spoon, spread into an even layer.

7. Cook for about 2–3 minutes.

8. Carefully, flip the side and cook for about 1 minute.

9. Repeat with the remaining mixture.

10. Serve warm with the drizzling of honey.

Preparation time: 15 minutes
Cooking time: 24 minutes
Total time: 39 minutes
Servings: 6

Nutritional Values

- Calories 232
- Total Fat 4.6 g
- Saturated Fat 0.6 g
- Cholesterol 0 mg
- Sodium 56 mg
- Total Carbs 46.3 g
- Fiber 5.3 g
- Sugar 16.2 g
- Protein 6 g

Smoked Salmon & Kale Scramble

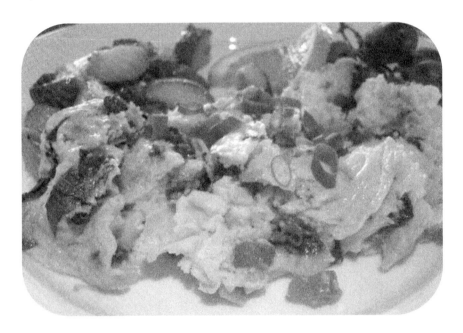

Ingredients

- 2 cups fresh kale, tough ribs removed and chopped finely
- 1 tablespoon coconut oil
- Ground black pepper, to taste
- ½ cup smoked salmon, crumbled
- 4 eggs, beaten

How to Prepare

1. In a wok, melt the coconut oil over high heat and cook the kale with black pepper for about 3–4 minutes.

2. Stir in the smoked salmon and reduce the heat to medium.
3. Add the eggs and cook for about 3–4 minutes, stirring frequently.
4. Serve immediately.

Preparation time: 10 minutes
Cooking time: 9 minutes
Total time: 19 minutes
Servings: 3

Nutritional Values

➢ Calories 257
➢ Total Fat 17 g
➢ Saturated Fat 8.9 g
➢ Cholesterol 335 mg
➢ Sodium 419 mg
➢ Total Carbs 7.7 g
➢ Fiber 1 g
➢ Sugar 0.7 g
➢ Protein 19.3 g

Kale & Mushroom Frittata

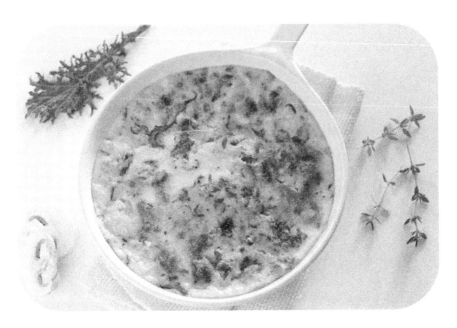

Ingredients

- ➤ 8 eggs
- ➤ ½ cup unsweetened almond milk
- ➤ Salt and ground black pepper, to taste
- ➤ 1 tablespoon olive oil
- ➤ 1 onion, chopped
- ➤ 1 garlic clove, minced
- ➤ 1 cup fresh mushrooms, chopped
- ➤ 1½ cups fresh kale, tough ribs removed and chopped

How to Prepare:

1. Preheat oven to 350°F.

2. In a large bowl, place the eggs, coconut milk, salt, and black pepper, and beat well. Set aside.

3. In a large ovenproof wok, heat the oil over medium heat and sauté the onion and garlic for about 3–4 minutes.

4. Add the squash, kale, bell pepper, salt, and black pepper, and cook for about 8–10 minutes.

5. Stir in the mushrooms and cook for about 3–4 minutes.

6. Add the kale and cook for about 5 minutes.

7. Place the egg mixture on top evenly and cook for about 4 minutes, without stirring.

8. Transfer the wok in the oven and bake for about 12–15 minutes or until desired doneness.

9. Remove from the oven and place the frittata side for about 3–5 minutes before serving.

10. Cut into desired sized wedges and serve.

Preparation time: 15 minutes
Cooking time: 30 minutes
Total time: 45 minutes
Servings: 5

Nutritional Values

- Calories 151
- Total Fat 10.2 g
- Saturated Fat 2.6 g
- Cholesterol 262 mg
- Sodium 158 mg
- Total Carbs 5.6 g
- Fiber 1 g
- Sugar 1.7 g
- Protein 10.3 g

Kale, Apple, & Cranberry Salad

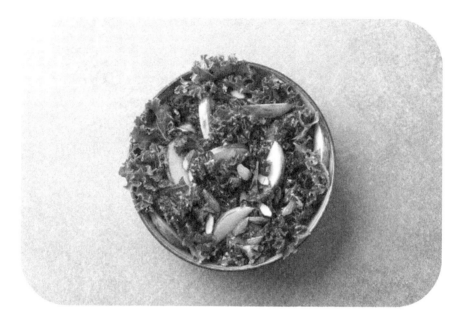

Ingredients

- ➢ 6 cups fresh baby kale
- ➢ 3 large apples, cored and sliced
- ➢ ¼ cup unsweetened dried cranberries
- ➢ ¼ cup almonds, sliced
- ➢ 2 tablespoons extra-virgin olive oil
- ➢ 1 tablespoon raw honey
- ➢ Salt and ground black pepper, to taste

How to Prepare:

1. In a salad bowl, place all the ingredients and toss to coat well.
2. Serve immediately.

Preparation time: 15 minutes
Total time: 15 minutes
Servings: 4

Nutritional Values

- ➢ *Calories 253*
- ➢ *Total Fat 10.3 g*
- ➢ *Saturated Fat 1.2 g*
- ➢ *Cholesterol 0 mg*
- ➢ *Sodium 84 mg*
- ➢ *Total Carbs 40.7 g*
- ➢ *Fiber 6.6 g*
- ➢ *Sugar 22.7 g*
- ➢ *Protein 4.7 g*

Arugula, Strawberry, & Orange Salad

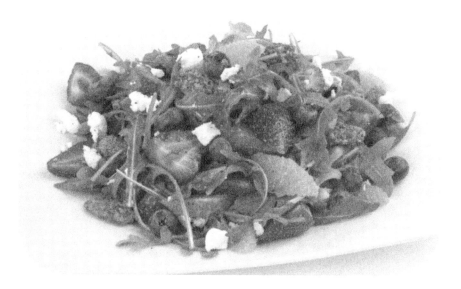

Ingredients

Salad
- 6 cups fresh baby arugula
- 1½ cups fresh strawberries, hulled and sliced
- 2 oranges, peeled and segmented

Dressing
- 2 tablespoons fresh lemon juice
- 1 tablespoon raw honey
- 2 teaspoons extra-virgin olive oil

- ➢ 1 teaspoon Dijon mustard
- ➢ Salt and ground black pepper, to taste

How to Prepare

1. For salad: in a salad bowl, place all ingredients and mix.
2. For dressing: place all ingredients in another bowl and beat until well combined.
3. Place dressing on top of salad and toss to coat well.
4. Serve immediately.

Preparation time: 15 minutes

Total time: 15 minutes

Servings: 4

Nutritional Values

- ➢ *Calories 107*
- ➢ *Total Fat 2.9 g*
- ➢ *Saturated Fat 0.4 g*
- ➢ *Cholesterol 0 mg*
- ➢ *Sodium 63 mg*
- ➢ *Total Carbs 20.6 g*
- ➢ *Fiber 3.9 g*
- ➢ *Sugar 16.4 g*
- ➢ *Protein 2.1 g*

Beef & Kale Salad

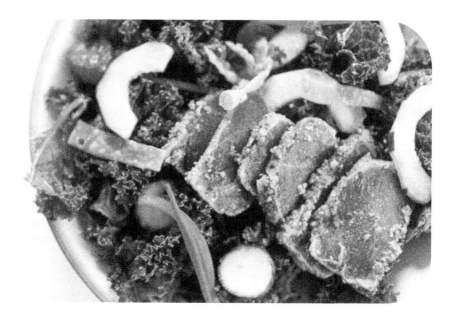

Ingredients

Steak
- ➢ 2 teaspoons olive oil
- ➢ 2 (4-ounce) strip steaks
- ➢ Salt and ground black pepper, to taste

Salad
- ➢ ¼ cup carrot, peeled and shredded
- ➢ ¼ cup cucumber, peeled, seeded, and sliced
- ➢ ¼ cup radish, sliced
- ➢ ¼ cup cherry tomatoes, halved
- ➢ 3 cups fresh kale, tough ribs removed and chopped

Dressing

- ➤ 1 tablespoon extra-virgin olive oil
- ➤ 1 tablespoon fresh lemon juice
- ➤ Salt and ground black pepper, to taste

How to Prepare

1. For steak: in a large heavy-bottomed wok, heat the oil over high heat and cook the steaks with salt and black pepper for about 3–4 minutes per side.
2. Transfer the steaks onto a cutting board for about 5 minutes before slicing.
3. For salad: place all ingredients in a salad bowl and mix.
4. For dressing: place all ingredients in another bowl and beat until well combined.
5. Cut the steaks into desired sized slices against the grain.
6. Place the salad onto each serving plate.
7. Top each plate with steak slices.
8. Drizzle with dressing and serve.

Preparation time: 15 minutes

Cooking time: 8 minutes

Total time: 23 minutes

Servings: 2

Nutritional Values

- Calories 262
- Total Fat 12 g
- Saturated Fat 1.6 g
- Cholesterol 63 mg
- Sodium 506 mg
- Total Carbs 15.2 g
- Fiber 2.5g
- Sugar 3.3 g
- Protein 25.2 g

Salmon Burgers

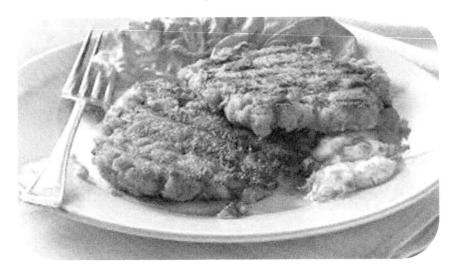

Ingredients

Burgers

- ➤ 1 teaspoon olive oil
- ➤ 1 cup fresh kale, tough ribs removed and chopped
- ➤ 1/3 cup shallots, chopped finely
- ➤ Salt and ground black pepper, to taste
- ➤ 16 ounces skinless salmon fillets
- ➤ ¾ cup cooked quinoa
- ➤ 2 tablespoons Dijon mustard
- ➤ 1 large egg, beaten

Salad

- ➢ 2½ tablespoons olive oil
- ➢ 2½ tablespoons red wine vinegar
- ➢ Salt and ground black pepper, to taste
- ➢ 8 cups fresh baby arugula
- ➢ 2 cups cherry tomatoes, halved

How to Prepare

1. For burgers: in a large non-stick wok, heat the oil over medium heat and sauté the kale, shallots, salt, and black pepper for about 4–5 minutes.
2. Remove from heat and transfer the kale mixture into a large bowl.
3. Set aside to cool slightly.
4. With a knife, chop 4 ounces of salmon and transfer into the bowl of kale mixture.
5. In a food processor, add the remaining salmon and pulse until finely chopped.
6. Transfer the finely chopped salmon into the bowl of kale mixture.
7. Then, add remaining ingredients and stir until fully combined.
8. Make 5 equal-sized patties from the mixture.

9. Heat a lightly greased large non-stick wok over medium heat and cook the patties for about 4–5 minutes per side.

10. For dressing: in a glass bowl, add the oil, vinegar, shallots, salt, and black pepper, and beat until well combined.

11. Add arugula and tomatoes and toss to coat well.

12. Divide the salad onto on serving plates and top each with 1 patty.

13. Serve immediately.

Preparation time: 20 minutes

Cooking time: 15 minutes

Total time: 35 minutes

Servings: 5

Nutritional Values

- *Calories 329*
- *Total Fat 15.8 g*
- *Saturated Fat 2.4 g*
- *Cholesterol 77 mg*
- *Sodium 177 mg*
- *Total Carbs 24 g*
- *Fiber 3.6 g*
- *Sugar 2.7 g*
- *Protein 24.9 g*

Chicken with Broccoli & Mushrooms

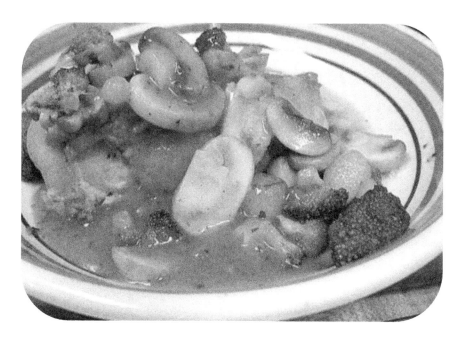

Ingredients

- 3 tablespoons olive oil
- 1 pound skinless, boneless chicken breast, cubed
- 1 medium onion, chopped
- 6 garlic cloves, minced
- 2 cups fresh mushrooms, sliced
- 16 ounces small broccoli florets
- ¼ cup water
- Salt and ground black pepper, to taste

How to Prepare

1. Heat the oil in a large wok over medium heat and cook the chicken cubes for about 4–5 minutes.
2. With a slotted spoon, transfer the chicken cubes onto a plate.
3. In the same wok, add the onion and sauté for about 4–5 minutes.
4. Add the mushrooms and cook for about 4–5 minutes.
5. Stir in the cooked chicken, broccoli, and water, and cook (covered) for about 8–10 minutes, stirring occasionally.
6. Stir in salt and black pepper and remove from heat.
7. Serve hot.

Preparation time: 15 minutes
Cooking time: 25 minutes
Total time: 40 minutes
Servings: 6

Nutritional Values

➢ *Calories 197*
➢ *Total Fat 10.1 g*
➢ *Saturated Fat 2 g*
➢ *Cholesterol 44 mg*
➢ *Sodium 82 mg*
➢ *Total Carbs 8.5 g*
➢ *Fiber 2.7 g*
➢ *Sugar 2.5 g*
➢ *Protein 20.1 g*

Beef with Kale & Carrot

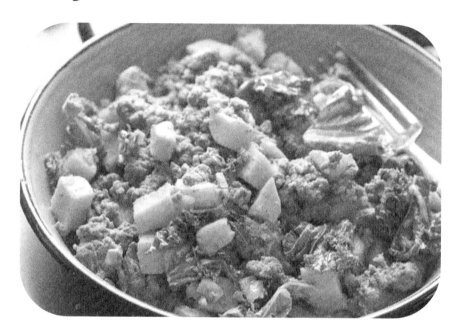

Ingredients

- 2 tablespoons coconut oil
- 4 garlic cloves, minced
- 1 pound beef sirloin steak, cut into bite-sized pieces
- Ground black pepper, to taste
- 1½ cups carrots, peeled and cut into matchsticks
- 1½ cups fresh kale, tough ribs removed and chopped
- 3 tablespoons tamari

How to Prepare

1. Melt the coconut oil in a wok over medium heat and sauté the garlic for about 1 minute.

2. Add the beef and black pepper and stir to combine.

3. Increase the heat to medium-high and cook for about 3–4 minutes or until browned from all sides.

4. Add the carrot, kale, and tamari, and cook for about 4–5 minutes.

5. Remove from the heat and serve hot.

Preparation time: 15 minutes

Cooking time: 12 minutes

Total time: 27 minutes

Servings: 4

Nutritional Values

➢ *Calories 311*
➢ *Total Fat 13.8 g*
➢ *Saturated Fat 8.6 g*
➢ *Cholesterol 101 mg*
➢ *Sodium 700 mg*
➢ *Total Carbs 8.4 g*
➢ *Fiber 1.6 g*
➢ *Sugar 2.3 g*
➢ *Protein 37.1 g*

Lamb Chops with Kale

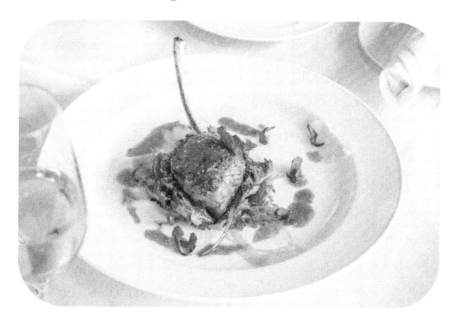

Ingredients

- ➢ 1 garlic clove, minced
- ➢ 1 tablespoon fresh rosemary leaves, minced
- ➢ Salt and ground black pepper, to taste
- ➢ 4 lamb loin chops
- ➢ 4 cups fresh baby kale

How to Prepare

1. Preheat the grill to high heat. Grease the grill grate.
2. In a bowl, add the garlic, rosemary, salt, and black pepper, and mix well.

3. Coat the lamb chops with the herb mixture generously.
4. Place the chops onto the hot side of grill and cook for about 2 minutes per side.
5. Now, move the chops onto the cooler side of the grill and cook for about 6–7 minutes.
6. Divide the kale onto serving plates and top each with 1 chop and serve.

Preparation time: 15 minutes
Cooking time: 11 minutes
Total time: 26 minutes
Servings: 4

Nutritional Values

➢ *Calories 301*
➢ *Total Fat 10.5 g*
➢ *Saturated Fat 3.8 g*
➢ *Cholesterol 128 mg*
➢ *Sodium 176 mg*
➢ *Total Carbs 7.8 g*
➢ *Fiber 1.4 g*
➢ *Sugar 0 g*
➢ *Protein 41.9 g*

Shrimp with Broccoli & Carrot

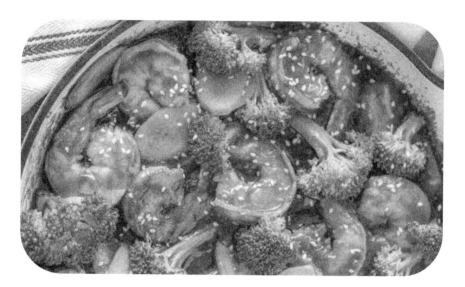

Ingredients

Sauce

- 1 tablespoon fresh ginger, grated
- 2 garlic cloves, minced
- 3 tablespoons low-sodium soy sauce
- 1 tablespoon red wine vinegar
- 1 teaspoon brown sugar
- ¼ teaspoon red pepper flakes, crushed

Shrimp Mixture

- 3 tablespoons olive oil
- 1½ pounds medium shrimp, peeled and deveined

119

- 12 ounces broccoli florets
- 8 ounces, carrot, peeled, and sliced

How to Prepare
1. For sauce: in a bowl, place all the ingredients and beat until well combined. Set aside.
2. In a large wok, heat oil over medium-high heat and cook the shrimp for about 2 minutes, stirring occasionally.
3. Add the broccoli and carrot and cook about 3–4 minutes, stirring frequently.
4. Stir in the sauce mixture and cook for about 1–2 minutes.
5. Serve immediately.

Preparation time: 15 minutes
Cooking time: 8 minutes
Total time: 23 minutes
Servings: 5

Nutritional Values
- *Calories 298*
- *Total Fat 10.7 g*
- *Saturated Fat 1.3 g*
- *Cholesterol 305 mg*
- *Sodium 882 mg*
- *Total Carbs 7 g*
- *Fiber 2g*
- *Sugar 2.4 g*
- *Protein 45.5 g*

Kale with Carrot

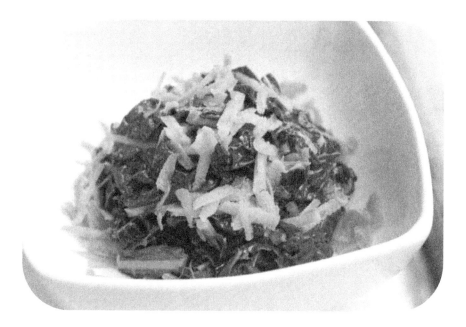

Ingredients

- ➢ 2 tablespoons olive oil
- ➢ 1 small onion, chopped
- ➢ 3 garlic cloves, minced
- ➢ 1 pound fresh kale, tough ribs removed and chopped
- ➢ ½ pound carrot, peeled and shredded
- ➢ 1 tablespoon raw honey
- ➢ 1 tablespoon fresh lemon juice
- ➢ Salt and ground black pepper, to taste

How to Prepare

1. Heat the oil in a large wok over medium heat and sauté the onion or about 4–5 minutes.

2. Stir in the garlic and sauté for about 1 minute.

3. Add the kale and cook for about 3–4 minutes.

4. Stir in the carrot, honey, lemon juice, salt, and black pepper, and cook for about 4–5 minutes.

5. Serve hot.

Preparation time: 15 minutes

Cooking time: 15 minutes

Total time: 30 minutes

Servings: 4

Nutritional Values

➢ *Calories 166*

➢ *Total Fat 7.1 g*

➢ *Saturated Fat 1 g*

➢ *Cholesterol 0 mg*

➢ *Sodium 129 mg*

➢ *Total Carbs 24.2 g*

➢ *Fiber 3.5 g*

➢ *Sugar 7.9 g*

➢ *Protein 4.2 g*

Chickpea with Swiss Chard

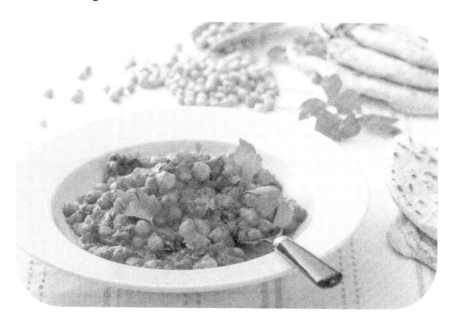

Ingredients

- 2 tablespoon olive oil
- 2 garlic cloves, sliced thinly
- 1 large tomato, chopped finely
- 2 bunches fresh Swiss chard, trimmed
- 1 (18-ounce) can chickpeas, drained and rinsed
- Salt and ground black pepper, to taste
- ¼ cup water
- 1 tablespoon fresh lemon juice
- 2 tablespoons fresh parsley, chopped

How to Prepare

1. Heat the oil in a large wok over medium heat and sauté the garlic for about 1 minute.
2. Add the tomato and cook for about 2–3 minutes, crushing with the back of spoon.
3. Stir in remaining ingredients except lemon juice and parsley and cook for about 5–7 minutes.
4. Drizzle with the lemon juice and remove from the heat.
5. Serve hot with the garnishing of parsley.

Preparation time: 15 minutes
Cooking time: 12 minutes
Total time: 27 minutes
Servings: 4

Nutritional Values

- *Calories 217*
- *Total Fat 8.3 g*
- *Saturated Fat 1 g*
- *Cholesterol 0 mg*
- *Sodium 171 mg*
- *Total Carbs 26.2 g*
- *Fiber 6.6 g*
- *Sugar 1.8 g*
- *Protein 8.8 g*

Beans & Kale Soup

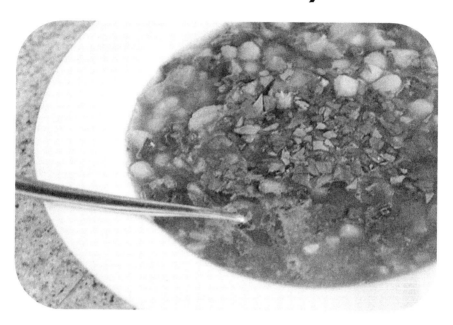

Ingredients

- ➢ 2 tablespoons olive oil
- ➢ 2 onions, chopped
- ➢ 4 garlic cloves, minced
- ➢ 1 pound kale, tough ribs removed and chopped
- ➢ 2 (14-ounce) cans cannellini beans, rinsed and drained
- ➢ 6 cups water
- ➢ Salt and ground black pepper, to taste

How to Prepare

1. In a large pan, heat the oil over medium heat and sauté the onion and garlic for about 4–5 minutes.

2. Add the kale and cook for about 1–2 minutes.
3. Add beans, water, salt, and black pepper, and bring to a boil.
4. Cook, partially covered for about 15–20 minutes.
5. Serve hot.

Preparation time: 15 minutes
Cooking time: 30 minutes
Total time: 45 minutes
Servings: 6

Nutritional Values

- *Calories 204*
- *Total Fat 4.7 g*
- *Saturated Fat 0.7 g*
- *Cholesterol 0 mg*
- *Sodium 85 mg*
- *Total Carbs 31.6 g*
- *Fiber 12.8 g*
- *Sugar 1.6 g*
- *Protein 11.5 g*

Tofu & Broccoli Curry

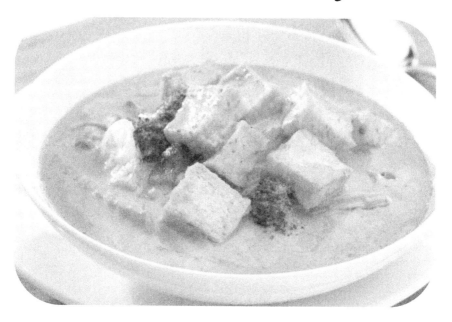

Ingredients

- ➤ 1 (16-ounce) block firm tofu, drained, pressed, and cut into ½-inch cubes
- ➤ 2 tablespoons coconut oil
- ➤ 1 medium yellow onion, chopped
- ➤ 1½ tablespoons fresh ginger, minced
- ➤ 2 garlic cloves, minced
- ➤ 1 tablespoon curry powder
- ➤ Salt and ground black pepper, to taste
- ➤ 1 cup fresh mushrooms, sliced
- ➤ 1 cup carrots, peeled and sliced
- ➤ 1 (14-ounce) can unsweetened low-fat coconut milk

- ½ cup low-sodium vegetable broth
- 2 teaspoons light brown sugar
- 10 ounces broccoli florets
- 1 tablespoon fresh lime juice
- ¼ cup fresh basil leaves, sliced thinly

How to Prepare

1. In a Dutch oven, heat the oil over medium heat and sauté the onion, ginger and garlic for about 5 minutes.

2. Stir in the curry powder, salt, and black pepper, and cook for about 2 minutes, stirring occasionally.

3. Add the mushrooms and carrot and cook for about 4–5 minutes.

4. Stir in the coconut milk, broth, and brown sugar, and bring to a boil.

5. Add the tofu and broccoli and simmer for about 12–15 minutes, stirring occasionally.

6. Stir in the lime juice and remove from the heat.

7. Serve hot.

Preparation time: 20 minutes

Cooking time: 30 minutes

Total time: 50 minutes

Servings: 5

Nutritional Values

- Calories 184
- Total Fat 11.1 g
- Saturated Fat 6.9 g
- Cholesterol 0 mg
- Sodium 55 mg
- Total Carbs 14.3 g
- Fiber 4.5 g
- Sugar 5 g
- Protein 10.5 g

Chicken & Veggies with Buckwheat Noodles

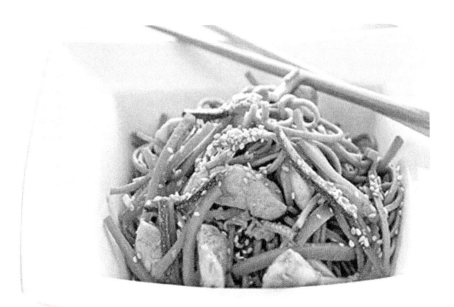

Ingredients

- ½ cup broccoli florets
- ½ cup fresh green beans, trimmed and sliced
- 1 cup fresh kale, tough ribs removed and chopped
- 5 ounces buckwheat noodles
- 1 tablespoon coconut oil
- 1 brown onion, chopped finely
- 1 (6-ounce) boneless, skinless chicken breast, cubed
- 2 garlic cloves, chopped finely
- 3 tablespoons low-sodium soy sauce

How to Prepare

1. In a medium pan of the boiling water, add the broccoli and green beans and cook for about 4–5 minutes.

2. Add the kale and cook for about 1–2 minutes.

3. Drain the vegetables and transfer into a large bowl. Set aside.

4. In another pan of the lightly salted boiling water, cook the soba noodles for about 5 minutes.

5. Drain the noodles well and then, rinse under cold running water. Set aside.

6. Meanwhile, in a large wok, melt the coconut oil over medium heat and sauté the onion for about 2–3 minutes.

7. Add the chicken cubes and cook for about 5–6 minutes.

8. Add the garlic, soy sauce and a little splash of water and cook for about 2–3 minutes, stirring frequently.

9. Add the cooked vegetables and noodles and cook for about 1–2 minutes, tossing frequently.

10. Serve hot with the garnishing of sesame seeds.

Preparation time: 20 minutes
Cooking time: 25 minutes
Total time: 45 minutes
Servings: 2

Nutritional Values

- Calories 463
- Total Fat 11.7 g
- Saturated Fat 5.9 g
- Cholesterol 54 mg
- Sodium 1000 mg
- Total Carbs 58.9 g
- Fiber 7.1 g
- Sugar 4.6 g
- Protein 22.5 g

Chocolate Muffins

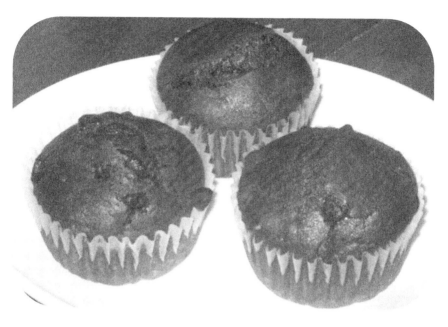

Ingredients

- ½ cup buckwheat flour
- ½ cup almond flour
- 4 tablespoons arrowroot powder
- 4 tablespoons cacao powder
- 1 teaspoon baking powder
- ½ teaspoon bicarbonate soda
- ½ cup boiled water
- 1/3 cup maple syrup
- 1/3 cup coconut oil, melted

- ➤ 1 tablespoon apple cider vinegar
- ➤ ½ cup unsweetened dark chocolate chips

How to Prepare

1. Preheat your oven to 350°F. Line 6 cups of a muffin tin with paper liners.
2. In a bowl, place the flours, arrowroot powder, baking powder, and bicarbonate of soda, and mix well.
3. In a separate bowl, place the boiled water, maple syrup, and coconut oil, and beat until well combined.
4. Now, place the flour mixture and mix until just combined.
5. Gently, fold in the chocolate chips.
6. Transfer the mixture into prepared muffin cups evenly.
7. Bake for about 20 minutes, or until a toothpick inserted in the center comes out clean.
8. Remove the muffin tin from oven and place onto a wire rack to cool for about 10 minutes.
9. Carefully invert the muffins onto the wire rack to cool completely before serving.

Preparation time: 15 minutes
Cooking time: 20 minutes
Total time: 35 minutes
Servings: 6

Nutritional Values

- *Calories 410*
- *Total Fat 28.6 g*
- *Saturated Fat 17.8 g*
- *Cholesterol 0 mg*
- *Sodium 25 mg*
- *Total Carbs 32.5 g*
- *Fiber 5.8 g*
- *Sugar 11.1 g*
- *Protein 4.6 g*

7-Day Meal Plan

Day 1

Breakfast: Matcha Green Juice

Lunch: Chicken, Kale, & Carrot Salad

Dinner: Lentils & greens Soup

Day 2

Breakfast: Kale Scramble

Lunch: Salmon Burgers

Dinner: Tofu & Broccoli Curry

Day 3

Breakfast: Blueberry Muffins

Lunch: Bok Choy & Mushroom Stir Fry

Dinner: Lamb Chops with Kale

Day 4

Breakfast: Buckwheat Granola

Lunch: Arugula, Strawberry, & Orange Salad

Dinner: Shrimp with Kale

Day 5

Breakfast: Broccoli, Apple, & Orange Juice

Lunch: Arugula & Berries Salad

Dinner: Chicken & Veggies with Buckwheat Noodles

Day 6

Breakfast: Matcha Pancakes

Lunch: Chickpeas with Swiss Chard

Dinner: Beef & Kale Salad

Day 7

Breakfast: Chocolate Waffles

Lunch: Rocket & Orange Salad

Dinner: Prawns with Asparagus

Conclusion

Now that you know sirtuins and their role better, following the sirtfood diet shouldn't be that difficult. Right? The diet has many more health benefits to guarantee then we can think of you. The rise in sirtuins in the body has been linked with a number of regulatory processes which indirectly leads to weight loss, active and healthy metabolism, etc. With the aim of turning your weight loss dream into a reality, this cookbook is designed to help you in the process through the good use of a sirtfood diet. All the recipes are created with sirtuin-rich food and they are equipped with easy to follow instructions. Let's give them a try and experience the ultimate benefits of a sirtfood diet!

Printed in Great Britain
by Amazon